Beyond The Body

Rethinking Weight
Reframing Health

By

Michael E. Hairston

TABLE OF CONTENTS

INTRODUCTION

Considering that our lives are inextricably intertwined with the threads of modernity, the impending epidemic of obesity has arisen as a ubiquitous and significant concern in this world. The book "Beyond the Body: Rethinking Weight, Reframing Health" dives deeply into the myriad of facets that comprise this worldwide health problem. It investigates the meaning of the crisis, its impact on individuals and societies, and the complex web of variables that contribute to its unrelenting ascent.

As we embark on this journey, it becomes increasingly clear that obesity is not only a matter of individual decisions or a singular health risk. It is a phenomenon that is both dynamic and complex, and it is profoundly ingrained in the fabric of our society, environment, genetics, and socioeconomic institutions. This book presents a detailed investigation that goes beyond the surface and covers the core causes and systemic implications of obesity. Its goal is to unravel the complicated tapestry that surrounds obesity.

In addition to this, the book investigates the profound psychological aspects of obesity, focusing on the complex relationship that exists between emotional well-being, stress, and eating behaviors. In this book, we look into the ways in which cultural standards, the influence of the media, and self-perception all contribute to a complicated narrative that molds individuals' relationships with their bodies and the dietary choices they make.

Furthermore, we investigate the systemic effects that obesity has on healthcare systems, economies, and social structures. This is in addition to the personal toll that obesity exacts on individuals. As we progress through the chapters of "Beyond the Body," readers will not only acquire a thorough comprehension of the complexities that are associated with obesity, but they will also acquire a revitalized sense of empathy for people who are struggling with this medical condition. In order to encourage meaningful conversations, raise awareness, and catalyze good change on both the individual and societal levels. As we travel the paths of understanding, compassion, and collective action in the face of the tremendous battle that characterizes our day, we invite you to join us on this illuminating adventure.

CHAPTER ONE

DEFINING OBESITY

A medical condition known as obesity is characterized by an excessive buildup of body fat, which results in an individual having a body mass index (BMI) of 30 or more. Obesity is a complication of obesity. The body mass index (BMI) of an individual can be determined by dividing their weight in kilograms by the square of their height in meters. Despite the fact that the body mass index (BMI) is a widely used indicator, it does not directly assess the proportion or distribution of body fat and may not appropriately reflect the health state of an individual.

There are numerous definitions and classifications of obesity, which take into account aspects such as body mass index (BMI), waist circumference, and the ratio of the waist to the hips. Based on the ranges of body mass index (BMI), the World Health Organization (WHO) categorizes obesity as follows: overweight from 25 to 29.9, obesity class I from 30 to 34.9, obesity class II from 35 to 39.9, and obesity class III from 40 or higher.

Over the course of the last few decades, the impact of obesity on the health of people all over the world has considerably increased, turning it into a major public health concern. There is a correlation between it and an increased risk of a variety of health illnesses, such as cardiovascular diseases, type 2 diabetes, some malignancies, musculoskeletal disorders, and psychological problems. Despite the fact that obesity is prominent in nations with high incomes, it has also grown increasingly common in countries with low and intermediate incomes, which contributes to the burden of non-communicable diseases that are experienced all over the world.

The correlation between obesity and a shorter life expectancy and a lower quality of life is a significant factor that highlights the importance of obesity as a social and health problem. There is a significant influence on the economy, as the costs of healthcare associated with obesity are putting pressure on healthcare systems all over the world. Comprehensive prevention and intervention techniques are required because of the intricate interaction of genetic, environmental, and behavioral factors that contribute to obesity.

It is necessary to take a diverse approach in order to combat obesity. This approach should include encouraging healthy dietary choices, increasing physical activity, and establishing circumstances that are helpful. In order to effectively battle the obesity pandemic, it is necessary to implement important components such as public health campaigns, regulatory changes, and community efforts. In order to establish methods that are both effective and equitable in addressing this global health concern, it is essential to acknowledge the social factors that contribute to obesity, such as access to education, employment, and healthcare.

CHAPTER 2

UNDERSTANDING THE CAUSES

The condition known as obesity is a complicated one that is formed by the intricate interaction of a number of different elements, each of which influences and interacts with the others. One of the key causes is diet, with the present prevalence of foods that are highly processed, high in caloric density, and rich in sugars and fats. It is possible for poor dietary habits, which are frequently formed by the ease with which certain items may be obtained, to result in an excessive consumption of calories and contribute to weight gain.

One of the most important contributors to the obesity pandemic is lifestyle factors. The reduction in physical activity that occurs as a consequence of sedentary behaviors is a direct effect of modern comforts such as desk jobs, vehicles, and entertainment based on screens. When combined with the prevalence of processed foods, this lack of physical activity creates an environment that is conducive to the accumulation of excess weight. The symbiotic relationship that exists between inactive lifestyles and bad dietary patterns creates a cycle that reinforces itself, hence increasing the likelihood of being overweight or obese.

Furthermore, genetics play a crucial role in determining an individual's likelihood of being overweight or obese. Despite the fact that genetic factors alone do not determine obesity, they can have an effect on the rate of metabolism, the storage of fat, and the regulation of appetite. It is possible that some genetic predispositions make certain persons more prone to gaining weight, particularly when they are exposed to an environment that is susceptible to obesity.

One of the most important elements that determine obesity is the environment, which includes things like the availability of healthy food selections and possibilities for physical activity. The availability of resources is frequently determined by socioeconomic differences; for example, persons with lower incomes face obstacles in gaining access to fresh, nutritious foods and secure areas for physical activity. The fact that there is a correlation between socioeconomic level and obesity highlights the importance of environmental factors in determining the outcomes of health care.

Societal factors, such as access to healthcare, career opportunities, and educational opportunities, are additional factors that contribute to the complexity of obesity. Educational access that is restricted may have an effect on nutritional understanding, and the conditions of employment may have an effect on the amount of time that is available for physical activity. It is possible that disparities in access to healthcare could have an impact on the quality of preventative and therapeutic measures, which would exacerbate health problems associated with obesity.

To get a complete understanding of obesity, it is necessary to acknowledge the interdependence of these elements. An example of this would be the interaction between genetic predispositions and an environment that is obesogenic, which would compound the risk for individuals. Furthermore, the socioeconomic determinants of obesity, which include education and employment, have the ability to impact lifestyle choices as well as access to healthcare, thereby generating a web of factors that together contribute to the development and continuation of obesity.

Interventions that take into consideration this complex interaction are required in order to address obesity in a comprehensive manner. The strategies should not only involve the modification of human behaviors but also the modification of structural aspects of the environment and the implementation of legislation that promotes health equity. When the multidimensional character of obesity is acknowledged, efforts can be focused on the creation of supportive environments that make it simpler for individuals from a variety of social and economic backgrounds to make choices that are healthy.

CHAPTER 3

MYTHS AND MISCONCEPTIONS

The stigma and discrimination that are associated with obesity are sometimes fueled by the myths and misconceptions that surround the condition. There is a widespread misconception that the only causes of obesity are a lack of self-control and excessive eating. This is an oversimplified view that is widely held. In actuality, the reasons that lead to obesity are multidimensional and include the complicated interplay between genetic, environmental, and behavioral factors. Because of this oversimplification, the physiological and psychological complications that people who are obese may experience are not taken into consideration.

The assumption that one's body weight is equivalent to one's overall health is yet another widespread fallacy. In some cases, being thin is not synonymous with being in good health, and being overweight is not necessarily a sign of being in poor health. The concept of health is intricate and multi-faceted, encompassing a wide range of aspects that go beyond weight. These aspects include nutrition, physical exercise, mental well-being, and genetic predispositions.

The assumption that people who are obese do not have the drive or ambition to change better lifestyles is a widespread myth that continues to be perpetuated. It is important to note that this oversimplification fails to take into account the difficulties that many individuals have in an environment that encourages bad eating choices and discourages physical activity. The formation of behaviors and decisions is also significantly influenced by a variety of elements, including socioeconomic conditions, psychological issues, and genetic factors.

Obesity is frequently linked to a moral character or personal value in attitudes that stigmatize the condition. This misunderstanding contributes to prejudice against people who are obese, which in turn has an effect on their experiences in social settings, professional settings, and healthcare settings. Obesity is not a reflection of an individual's character or value; rather, it is a complex health problem that should be recognized by those working in the healthcare industry, those who determine policy, and the general public.

When it comes to obesity, there is a common misunderstanding that weight loss is always a straightforward and efficient remedy. The process of losing weight is not a one-size-fits-all solution, despite the fact that it may be advantageous for certain people. There are a number of factors that can influence the success of weight loss efforts, including heredity, metabolism, and diseases that are present in the body. The major focus should be on promoting overall health through changes in lifestyle that are sustainable, regardless of whether or not there is a modification in weight.

Putting these myths to the test is absolutely necessary in order to cultivate empathy and comprehension. In order to avoid being counterproductive, it is vital to acknowledge that people who are obese may encounter specific obstacles when it comes to maintaining their weight. Blaming or stigmatizing these persons is unacceptable. The promotion of a more nuanced and evidence-based knowledge of obesity helps to contribute to the creation of a supportive atmosphere that fosters behaviors that are focused on health without perpetuating discrimination or bias.

CHAPTER 4

PHYSICAL HEALTH CONSEQUENCES

The condition of obesity is linked to a wide range of physical health issues, each of which has the potential to profoundly influence the well-being of an individual. Obesity is highly associated with a number of serious and widespread health problems, including cardiovascular disorders. People who have a higher body mass index are at a greater risk of developing cardiovascular diseases and conditions such as coronary artery disease, stroke, and arterial hypertension. The accumulation of fatty deposits in blood vessels and the increased stress placed on the heart are both factors that contribute to the development of cardiovascular problems at this time.

There is a strong correlation between obesity and type 2 diabetes, as having excess body fat might have an effect on insulin sensitivity. There is a correlation between obesity and insulin resistance, which can result in raised blood sugar levels and an increased likelihood of developing diabetes. The risk of cardiovascular disease is further increased by this chronic condition, which also has the potential to result in consequences such as kidney disease, nerve damage, and concerns regarding vision.

There is a correlation between obesity and an increased risk of developing some types of cancer. Obesity is linked to an increased chance of acquiring cancers such as breast, colorectal, ovarian, and pancreatic cancer. The intricate interactions that occur between adipose tissue, inflammation, and hormone variables are the mechanisms that are responsible for contributing to this connection.

Individuals who are obese are more likely to suffer from musculoskeletal diseases because of the increased mechanical stress that is placed on weight-bearing joints at this weight. As a result of the acceleration of joint degradation caused by excess body weight, conditions such as osteoarthritis are becoming increasingly widespread. In addition to back pain and gout, musculoskeletal problems that are commonly connected with obesity include reduced mobility and back discomfort.

Certain respiratory problems, such as sleep apnea, are becoming increasingly common as a result of obesity's effects on the respiratory system. The buildup of fat around the neck and throat region can be a consequence of having an excessive amount of body weight, which can contribute to the obstruction of the airway when sleeping. As a consequence, this causes disruptions in the patterns of breathing, which can result in exhaustion during the day as well as other difficulties.

Disorders of the gastrointestinal tract, such as gallbladder disease and fatty liver disease, are more prevalent in those who are obese. Non-alcoholic fatty liver disease, often known as NAFLD, is characterized by the buildup of fat in the liver. If the illness is not handled, it can proceed to more severe liver problems.

There is a significant influence that obesity has on the reproductive system, and this impact is seen in both males and females. A number of health problems, including menstruation abnormalities, infertility, and issues during pregnancy, have been linked to obesity in females. Men are susceptible to hormone imbalances that can have an impact on their fertility.

Individuals who are obese are at a greater risk of experiencing mental health issues such as sadness, anxiety, and low self-esteem. Obesity also has an impact on psychological well-being. The social stigma that is linked with obesity can be an additional factor that contributes to difficulties with mental health.

Overall, the effects of obesity on one's health are extensive and multi-faceted, and they are far-reaching. A complete approach that takes into consideration the prevention and management of associated health issues, as well as the promotion of overall well-being and the improvement of quality of life for those who are impacted by obesity, is required in order to address the issue of obesity. Controlling weight is only one component of this comprehensive approach.

CHAPTER 5

MENTAL AND EMOTIONAL HEALTH IMPLICATIONS

Beyond the negative effects that obesity has on one's physical health, it also has a wide range of psychological and emotional repercussions, which can have a variety of complex effects on one's mental well-being. One of the most prevalent mental health problems that is related to obesity is depression. The stigma and prejudice that individuals with obesity confront in society can contribute to feelings of social isolation, low self-esteem, and a sense of hopelessness. All of these are variables that can contribute to the development of depressive symptoms or to the exacerbation of existing symptoms.

Anxiety is another common mental health condition that is widespread among people who are obese. It is possible that increased levels of anxiety are caused by a combination of factors, including the pressure from society to conform to particular body ideals, as well as potential concerns for health and well-being. Another factor that may lead to social anxiety is the fear of being judged or of being perceived negatively by other people.

The environment of obesity is one in which difficulties pertaining to body image are especially prevalent. Individuals who are obese may internalize unfavorable thoughts about their bodies since societal ideals frequently place a priority on thinness that is considered desirable. This can result in a skewed perception of oneself, an obsession with one's physical appearance, and a detrimental effect on one's sense of self-worth. The development of unhealthy eating habits or disordered eating patterns may also be influenced by a person's dissatisfaction with their body or appearance.

In persons who are obese, the prevalence of eating disorders, such as binge eating disorder, is significantly higher. Disordered eating behaviors can be a contributing factor to the psychological distress that is associated with weight-related problems. This creates a complex interaction between mental health and obesity.

The emotional toll of obesity is not limited to the individual, but it also extends to the connections that people have with one another. People who are obese may be subjected to prejudice, discrimination, and judgment from other people, which can result in such individuals experiencing feelings of shame and social marginalization. This societal stigma has the potential to negatively impact personal relationships, the conditions in which people work, and the quality of life in general.

Furthermore, the cyclical nature of the interaction between mental and physical health in obesity can create a loop that is difficult to break. The cycle of mental and emotional difficulties can be perpetuated by psychological anguish, which can lead to poor coping techniques or excessive eating, which in turn can further exacerbate worries connected to weight and bring about other complications.

The mental and emotional health implications of obesity are an essential component of comprehensive care, and it is important to address these implications. Not only should a holistic approach include weight management measures, but it should also include psychological support, counseling, and treatments that are targeted at developing a positive self-image, self-acceptance, and enhanced mental well-being. In order to promote a more compassionate and effective response to the issues that persons who are coping with obesity confront, it is vital to acknowledge the interdependence of mental and physical health.

CHAPTER 6

SOCIOECONOMIC AND CULTURAL INFLUENCES

There is a considerable relationship between the socioeconomic and cultural elements that play a role in shaping the risk and prevalence of obesity. There is a strong correlation between socioeconomic position and obesity, with persons in lower-income groups being at a greater risk of being obese. When people living in low-income neighborhoods have limited access to affordable and nutritious food options, this can lead to an increase in the intake of processed foods that are rich in sugars and fats and are high in energy density. Additionally, persons with lower incomes may face financial challenges due to the high cost of fresh fruit and other dietary options that are healthier.

It is possible for cultural norms and values to have an effect on the risk of obesity in relation to food choices and eating behaviors. It is possible that traditional diets in certain cultures are high in foods that are high in calories, and that communal dining traditions may encourage portion sizes that are greater. It is common practice for cultural holidays and ceremonies to entail the consumption of specific delicacies, which might lead to excessive eating.

Additionally, the built environment, which is impacted by socioeconomic conditions, is a source of influence. It may be difficult for inhabitants of low-income neighborhoods to engage in regular exercise since there may not be enough safe locations for physical activity, such as parks or recreational facilities. As a result of the restricted availability of reasonably priced and nutritious food options, individuals may be forced to rely on the products of fast food restaurants or convenience stores.

It is possible that cultural attitudes on body weight and size can lead to worries about body image and potentially have an effect on the prevalence of obesity. Larger body sizes may be culturally accepted or even praised in some countries, yet in other cultures, there may be tremendous societal pressures to adhere to a particular body ideal. This can change depending on the culture. These cultural norms have the potential to influence individuals' perceptions of their bodies and may be a contributing factor in the formation of varied attitudes on fitness and weight.

Additionally, socioeconomic variables have the potential to impact educational opportunities and health literacy, which in turn can have an effect on understanding regarding nutrition and good lifestyle choices. There may be a lack of awareness about the significance of maintaining a healthy diet and engaging in physical activity due to limited access to appropriate educational opportunities.

As a result of the intersection of socioeconomic and cultural effects, there is a pressing requirement for interventions that are both individualized and sensitive to cultural norms in order to combat obesity. It is important for initiatives that attempt to promote healthier lifestyles to take into account the economic realities and cultural surroundings of the communities that they intend to serve. When making efforts to enhance access to inexpensive and nutritious foods, develop safe spaces for physical exercise, and promote health education, it is important to keep in mind the myriad of socioeconomic and cultural factors that contribute to the different levels of obesity that exist in different populations. The development of methods that are both effective and equitable in addressing the global challenge of obesity requires first and foremost an acknowledgment of the complexity of the variables at play.

CHAPTER 7

DEBUNKING DIET FADS

Despite the fact that fad diets often come with major limitations and hazards, they frequently promise to produce weight reduction results that are both rapid and dramatic. The absence of sustainability is a problem that frequently arises. Many of the diets that are currently popular are extremely restricted, either by omitting entire food groups or by imposing stringent calorie limits. Although it is possible that this will result in immediate weight loss, it is difficult to adhere to such restricted diets over an extended period of time, which frequently leads to the regaining of weight that was lost.

There is also the possibility that fad diets are deficient in important nutrients, which could result in nutritional deficits. Eating habits that are restrictive can cause the body to be deprived of essential vitamins, minerals, and macronutrients, which can have a negative impact on general health. In order to maintain a healthy weight, it is vital to consume a diet that is both well-balanced and diverse, and that supplies the essential nutrients for the body's processes.

Diets that are considered to be trendy frequently rely on anecdotal evidence or studies that have been selectively chosen, rather than being founded on solid scientific study. There is a possibility that specific success stories will be highlighted; nevertheless, these stories do not represent the variety of reactions that can be found among diverse people. A wide amount of scientific data is taken into consideration by evidence-based methods for healthy eating for weight management. These approaches also place a higher priority on long-term health outcomes than they do on short-term results.

Fad diets, which place a focus on rapid cures, can lead to unhealthy relationships with food if they are followed. It is possible that extreme dietary limitations could result in feelings of deprivation, guilt, or worry, all of which can contribute to disordered eating patterns for the individual. Eating healthily should encourage a constructive and long-term approach, with the primary emphasis being placed on nourishing the body rather than concentrating on achieving weight loss goals in the short term.

There is a tendency for fad diets to disregard the significance of individually tailored approaches to nutrition. Different metabolic rates, genetic factors, and lifestyle considerations all contribute to the fact that every individual's body is one of a kind. A method that is universally applicable does not take into account the individual differences that exist. Approaches to healthy eating that are supported by evidence take into account the specific requirements, preferences, and health objectives of each individual, so offering a more individualized and efficient method for managing weight over the long term.

In order to promote a holistic approach to healthy eating, it is necessary to take into consideration not only what to eat but also which foods to eat. In order to cultivate a good relationship with food, it is essential to engage in mindful eating habits. These activities include paying attention to indicators that indicate when you are hungry and when you are full, savoring flavors, and eating meals in an atmosphere that is comfortable. It is possible to achieve a sustainable and well-balanced approach to weight management by concentrating on making adjustments to one's lifestyle as a whole, which includes engaging in regular physical activity and learning how to manage stress.

As a conclusion, the process of debunking diet fads requires acknowledging the limits of these diets, which include their inability to be maintained over time, the possibility of nutritional inadequacies, their reliance on anecdotal evidence, and their promotion of quick remedies. On the other hand, advocating for evidence-based methods of healthy eating places an emphasis on long-term sustainability, nutritional balance, individualized tactics, and a holistic focus on total well-being.

CHAPTER 8

RETHINKING WEIGHT, REFRAMING HEALTH

When it comes to maintaining a healthy weight and general health, physical activity is of the utmost importance. Through the burning of calories and the improvement of metabolism, exercises that are performed on a regular basis contribute to weight loss and help maintain a healthy weight. Moreover, it has several advantages for the health of the cardiovascular system, the power of the muscles, the mental well-being, and the reduction of the risk of developing chronic diseases.

The incorporation of physical activity into daily routines is absolutely necessary for individuals who are interested in efficiently managing their weight. Taking the stairs instead of the lift, walking or biking to work, or implementing small bursts of physical activity throughout the day, such as stretching or fast exercises, can make a huge difference. These are just some of the simple techniques that can make a difference.

Walking, running, swimming, or cycling are examples of aerobic workouts. Strength training activities, such as lifting weights or exercises using only your own body weight, are examples of strength training activities. This mix of exercises is good for promoting general health and managing weight. Strength training helps build lean muscle mass, which boosts metabolism and allows for weight loss. Aerobic workouts help improve cardiovascular fitness and burn calories. Strength training also helps promote weight loss.

The ability to find physical activities that one enjoys is essential for maintaining commitment over the long run. Participating in activities that generate joy, such as dancing, hiking, playing a sport, or taking part in group fitness classes, enhances the likelihood that these activities will be incorporated into a regular routine.

Maintaining consistency is essential. In order to build a routine, it is helpful to set goals that are both attainable and practical. For example, one could strive to walk a certain number of steps every day or set aside a particular amount of time for a workout. Alterations that are both long-lasting and beneficial can be brought about by gradually increasing the intensity and duration of physical activity over the course of time.

The concept of incorporating movement into daily life encompasses more than just traditional exercise. Activities that are performed on a daily basis, such as gardening, performing chores around the house, or playing with pets, all add to the total levels of physical activity. In order to achieve this goal, mobility should become a natural part of daily life.

The advantages of physical activity extend far beyond the control of one's weight; it also has a significant impact on one's mental health. Endorphins are released during exercise, which helps reduce feelings of tension, anxiety, and symptoms of sadness. Enhancing one's mood, increasing one's energy levels, and improving one's general quality of life can all be accomplished by engaging in physical activity.

In addition, adding movement into social activities, such as going for a stroll with a buddy, joining a sports team, or attending group fitness classes, can add a social component to exercise, making it more fun and even more sustainable.

The aim of treating obesity is to get to and maintain a healthy weight. This enhances general health and reduces the likelihood of obesity-related problems.

To better understand and modify your food and exercise habits, you might need to collaborate with a group of medical specialists, such as a nutritionist, behavioral counselor, or obesity specialist.

Typically, the first treatment objective is to lose 5% to 10% of your body weight. This implies that for your health to start improving, you would only need to shed roughly 10 to 20 pounds (4.5 to 9 kilograms) if you weigh 200 pounds (91 kilograms). However, the advantages increase with the amount of weight lost.

Every weight-loss program calls on you to increase your physical activity and make dietary changes. Your weight, general health, and desire to follow a weight-loss plan will determine which therapy options are best for you.

Dietary adjustments

The secret to reducing obesity is cutting calories and adopting better eating practices. Even though you might lose weight quickly at initially, the safest strategy to reduce weight is to lose weight gradually over time. It's also the most effective approach to maintain weight loss over time. The ideal weight-loss diet does not exist. Select the one you think will work best for you, one that includes nutritious foods. Treatment options for obesity with diet include:

• **Reducing caloric intake:** The secret to losing weight is cutting back on your caloric intake. Examining your normal eating and drinking routines is the first step. You may check how many calories you typically eat and identify areas for reduction. How many calories you need to consume daily to lose weight is something you and your healthcare provider may determine together. For women, a typical serving size is 1,200–1,500 calories, while for men it is 1,500–1,800.

• **Feeling content yet less:** Certain foods, like sweets, candies, fats, and processed foods, have a high-calorie content per serving. Fruits and vegetables, on the other hand, offer a higher serving size with fewer calories. You can lessen food cravings and consume fewer calories by eating greater portions of lower-calorie items. Additionally, you can feel better about your food, which raises your level of satisfaction in general.

• **Selecting healthier options:** Eat more plant-based foods to improve the health of your diet as a whole. They consist of whole grains, fruits, and vegetables. Additionally, emphasize lean meats and other lean protein sources like soy, lentils, and beans. Try to eat fish twice a week if you enjoy it. Reduce your intake of salt and added sugar. Consume fats in moderation, and make sure they come from heart-healthy sources such as nuts, canola, and olive oils.

• **Limiting specific food groups:** Some diets place restrictions on the quantity of foods high in fat or carbohydrates. Find out from your healthcare provider which diets are beneficial to you and which are not. Consuming beverages with added sugar is a guaranteed method to eat more calories than you planned. A smart place to start when reducing your calorie intake is to limit or stop these drinks completely.

• **Meal replacements:** These plans advocate eating healthful snacks and substituting one or two meals a day with their goods, such as meal bars or low-calorie drinks. After that, you take a third meal that is low in calories and fat and is well-balanced. You can lose weight with this kind of diet in the short term. However, you probably won't learn how to alter your lifestyle in general from these diets. Thus, if you want to maintain your weight loss, you might need to stick to the diet.

Avoid using fast fixes. Fad diets that promise quick and simple weight loss may attract you. However, the truth is that neither miracle meals nor fast cures exist. Fad diets might be beneficial in the short run, but they don't seem to work much better in the long run than regular diets.

In a similar vein, while going on a crash diet could help you lose weight, you probably won't get it back afterwards. You need to develop long-lasting healthy eating habits if you want to lose weight and keep it off.

Activity and exercise

Increasing one's level of exercise or physical activity is crucial for treating obesity:

• **Exercise:** Individuals who suffer from obesity should engage in moderate-intense physical activity for at least 150 minutes each week. This can maintain weight loss or stop additional weight gain of a moderate amount. As your endurance and fitness improve, you'll probably need to progressively increase the amount of exercise you get in.

• **Don't stop moving:** Although frequent aerobic exercise is the most effective approach to burn calories and lose extra weight, any additional movement also contributes to calorie burning. Take the stairs rather than the elevator, for instance, and park further away from store entrances. You can keep track of how many steps you take each day with a pedometer. A lot of people attempt to walk 10,000 steps a day. Increase the amount of steps you take each day to accomplish your objective gradually.

Modifications in behavior

To lose weight and keep it off, you can modify your lifestyle with the support of a behavior modification program. One of the first things to do is to examine your existing routine to determine what stresses, circumstances, or other elements may have led to your obesity.

Therapy: Speaking with a mental health professional can assist in addressing behavioral and emotional eating-related concerns. You can acquire healthier coping mechanisms for anxiety and comprehend why you overeat with the support of therapy. Additionally, you can learn how to recognize eating triggers, keep an eye on your diet and exercise, and manage food cravings. Group or one-on-one counseling are both possible.

Support Teams: Friendships and understanding can be found in support groups where members deal with similar obesity-related issues. To find support groups in your area, ask your medical team, nearby hospitals, or for-profit weight-loss programs.

Medications for weight loss

Medication for weight loss should not be used in place of diet, exercise, and behavioral changes. Your healthcare provider will take into account potential side effects in addition to your medical history when choosing a medicine for you.

The most often prescribed drugs for treating obesity that have been approved by the Food and Drug Administration (FDA) in the United States are

Bupropion-naltrexone (Contrave)."

Astagliptide (Liraglutide).

Orlistat (Xenical, Alli).

Qsymia is phentermine-topiramate.

Semaglutide (Rybelsus, Wegovy, Ozempic). (Seek the help of a professional before taking these drugs)

Not everyone will benefit from weight-loss medications, and their effects may eventually wear off. You can gain back most or all of the weight you lose after you stop taking medication for weight loss.

Lifestyle choices and DIY solutions

If you incorporate at-home tactics into your formal treatment plan, your chances of overcoming obesity are increased. Educating yourself about your condition is one of these. You may discover more about the causes of your obesity and what you can do about it by becoming educated about the condition. You may feel more equipped to take charge and follow your treatment plan. Go through credible self-help books and think about discussing them with your therapist or medical expert.

• **Making sensible goals:** If you need to shed a lot of weight, you can make unreasonable objectives for yourself, including trying to reduce too much weight too quickly. Avoid positioning yourself for failure. Make fitness and weight loss objectives for each day or each week. Rather than trying to make big, unsustainable changes to your diet, start with little, manageable modifications.

• **Adhering to your treatment plan:** It might be challenging to alter a way of life that you have led for a long time. If you find that you are not meeting your exercise or dietary objectives, be honest with your doctor, therapist, or other health care providers. You can collaborate to generate fresh concepts or methods.

• **Recruiting assistance:** Recruit your friends and family to support your weight-loss efforts. Assemble a team of people who will aid and encourage you rather than undermine your efforts. Ensure that they comprehend the significance of losing weight for your well-being. Joining a support group for weight loss could also be beneficial.

• **Maintaining a log:** Maintain a food and exercise diary. You can hold yourself more responsible for your eating and exercise habits by keeping this diary. You can find out what might be preventing you from moving forward. You may also see what is most effective for you. You can monitor additional vital health indicators with your log, such as blood pressure, cholesterol, and general level of fitness.

CHAPTER 9

BEHAVIORAL AND PSYCHOLOGICAL STRATEGIES

Cognitive-behavioral therapy, sometimes known as CBT, is a popular form of psychological intervention that focuses on addressing the behavioral and psychological variables that contribute to harmful behaviors connected to weight. When it comes to weight management, cognitive behavioral therapy (CBT) focuses on recognizing and altering negative thought patterns and behaviors that are related to eating and physical activity. In addition to addressing the emotional elements that influence weight-related behaviors, it seeks to encourage healthy habits, boost self-esteem, and enhance overall health.

The process of identifying and addressing erroneous attitudes and beliefs regarding food, body image, and weight is an essential part of cognitive behavioral therapy (CBT). Through the process of learning to recognize and reframe negative self-talk, individuals are able to lessen the influence that unhelpful beliefs have on their behaviors. This cognitive restructuring assists in the development of an attitude that is more optimistic and grounded in reality towards food and the body.

The difficulty of emotional eating is a common one, and cognitive behavioral therapy (CBT) offers techniques to deal with feelings without resorting to food as a means of consolation. Improving one's emotional awareness and developing healthy coping strategies can be accomplished through the implementation of techniques such as mindfulness and stress management approaches.

In cognitive behavioral therapy (CBT), behavioral methods are utilized to manage impulsivity, which is frequently linked to poor eating behaviors. Individuals acquire the knowledge and skills necessary to execute behavioral methods, such as establishing certain objectives, preparing meals in advance, and establishing an atmosphere that encourages healthy decision-making. An organized approach to eating can be created with the help of these tactics, which also help reduce impulsivity.

In addition, cognitive behavioral therapy (CBT) investigates the connection between ideas, feelings, and behaviors, which assists clients in comprehending the factors that lead to harmful eating patterns. People can create alternate, healthier reactions to these triggers if they first identify the antecedents and effects of their actions and then work to develop such responses.

Both dialectical behavior therapy (DBT) and acceptance and commitment therapy (ACT) are examples of additional psychological interventions that are complementary to cognitive behavioral therapy (CBT). Individuals who are battling with emotional eating may benefit from dialectical behavior therapy (DBT) since it places an emphasis on developing skills in distress tolerance, emotion regulation, and interpersonal efficacy with other people. ACT is a form of psychotherapy that focuses on fostering psychological flexibility by assisting clients in accepting challenging thoughts and feelings while simultaneously committing to activities that are in line with their core beliefs.

Other methods that are frequently utilized to resolve ambivalence and boost the desire for behavior change include motivational interviewing and motivational counseling. It is possible for therapists to assist clients in overcoming resistance and developing a personalized strategy for healthy behaviors by conducting an investigation into the inner motivations, values, and goals of various individuals.

It has been found that therapies that are centered on families are particularly beneficial, particularly for children and adolescents. The family is involved in the process of building a supportive atmosphere that fosters healthy food and physical activity habits. These approaches come from the perspective of the family.

When it comes to tackling emotional eating, impulsivity, and other characteristics that contribute to unhealthy weight-related behaviors, cognitive-behavioral therapy and other psychological interventions play a significant role in addressing these issues. Individuals are provided with the tools necessary to shift negative thought patterns, cope with emotions in a more healthy manner, and execute behavior changes that support long-term weight control and overall well-being through the utilization of these tactics.

CHAPTER 10

PUBLIC HEALTH AND POLICY INTERVENTIONS

The creation of surroundings that encourage healthy lives is a crucial component in the fight against obesity, and public health initiatives and legislative changes are essential components in this fight. One of the most important focuses is on boosting nutrition education and awareness programs in order to educate the general population about the need to control portion sizes, make good food choices, and the influence that dietary habits have on overall health. The purpose of these programs is to provide individuals with the ability to make educated decisions regarding their nutrition and lifestyle choices.

The most important thing is to put into effect measures that will make food more accessible and affordable. This includes activities such as encouraging farmer's markets, improving the availability of fresh and nutritious foods in communities that are neglected, and providing incentives to grocery shops so that they carry better options. It is also possible for policy interventions to alleviate food deserts, which are regions that have inadequate access to food that is both affordable and healthy. This can be accomplished by encouraging the creation of grocery shops of community gardens.

In the realm of public health, campaigns and legislative changes frequently focus on reducing the amount of bad fats and added sugars that are included in processed foods. In order to assist customers in making better decisions, the implementation of clear and standardized nutritional labeling on food products is essential. Furthermore, policies that restrict the marketing of unhealthy foods to children can play a role in the development of healthier eating habits beginning at a younger age. Another important factor is encouraging people to engage in physical activity. Increasing the amount of daily mobility can be accomplished through the development of neighborhoods that are conducive to walking, the planning of urban environments that promote physical exercise, and the investment in public transit. Interventions that are implemented in schools, such as mandatory physical education classes and the provision of nutritious school meals, are extremely important in the process of molding the behaviors of young students.

By supporting wellness programs, giving incentives for physical activity, and fostering supportive work settings that encourage healthy eating, policy changes can be implemented to address the environment of the workplace. The implementation of workplace regulations that encourage a healthy balance between work and personal life can also contribute to a reduction in stress and an improvement in general well-being.

It is possible to use taxation laws as a tool to discourage the consumption of unhealthy foods and beverages, such as sugary drinks with high levels of sugar. Because of this, their affordability may diminish, which may ultimately lead to a reduction in their use. A similar effect can be achieved by providing subsidies for the production and promotion of healthier foods, which can make these foods more accessible and inexpensive for the general public.

There is a critical need for interventions that are carried out within schools. These interventions include the establishment of physical education programs and policies that restrict the sorts of meals and beverages that are offered in schools. The use of these strategies helps to establish an atmosphere that encourages the development of healthy behaviors at an early age.

In order for public health efforts to be successful, community engagement is an essential component. Through the participation of communities in the planning and execution of programs, it is possible to guarantee that interventions are sensitive to cultural norms and cater to the specific requirements of the community.

To summarise, the implementation of public health programs and the modification of policies are essential components in the fight against obesity because they produce environments that encourage healthy behaviors. These interventions address systemic concerns, contribute to the formation of social norms, and help to contribute to the establishment of a culture that supports and encourages individuals and communities to make healthy personal and community choices.

CHAPTER 11

BUILDING SUPPORTIVE COMMUNITIES

In order to cultivate surroundings that are conducive to weight control and overall well-being, supportive groups, which may include family, friends, and healthcare professionals, play an essential role.

In order for individuals to successfully manage their weight, having the support of their family is essential. The development of healthy food habits, regular physical activity, and mental well-being are all fostered by circumstances that are supportive of families. There is a supportive environment that may be created through activities such as eating together, going grocery shopping together, and participating in physical activities as a family. It is possible for members of the family to offer emotional support, understanding, and motivation, so establishing an atmosphere in which good behaviors are promoted and rewarded.

When it comes to keeping healthy behaviors, peer support is an important factor. The encouragement and accountability that can be provided by friends who have similar health goals is invaluable. Exercise can be made more fun and durable by participating in social activities that are centered around physical activity. Some examples of such activities include group workouts or sports. A sense of community and a shared commitment to one's well-being can be fostered through the provision of positive reinforcement and encouragement with the help of friends.

When it comes to offering counsel and assistance for weight management, healthcare experts, such as physicians, dietitians, and psychologists, play an essential role. They are able to provide individualized guidance on aspects such as fitness, diet, and behavior modification. Monitoring progress, addressing obstacles, and modifying tactics as required are all opportunities that can be taken advantage of during routine checkups. Furthermore, healthcare experts are able to assist clients in navigating the emotional aspects of weight management, thereby addressing the underlying psychological reasons that may contribute to unhealthy behaviors.

An atmosphere that is supportive is facilitated by programs and initiatives that are grounded in the community. Fitness courses, nutritional workshops, and support groups are some examples of these types of activities. These groups allow people who have similar aims to connect with one another and share their experiences. Participating in community activities helps to cultivate a sense of belonging and encourages collaborative efforts to lead healthy lives.

By instituting wellness programs in the workplace, employers have the ability to make a positive contribution to the overall atmosphere. Among them may be fitness competitions, campaigns to promote a healthy diet, and policies that encourage a good balance between work and personal life. Environments in the workplace that are supportive allow employees to put their health and wellness first and to make decisions that are better for them.

Additional factors that contribute to the formation of supportive settings include educational institutions and schools. The formation of good habits in young people is facilitated by the implementation of health education programs, the provision of nutritious school meals, and the mandated participation in physical education. Modeling healthy behaviors and providing positive reinforcement are two things that teachers and other school staff may do.

Through the promotion of positive body ideals, various portrayals of beauty, and messaging that encourages healthy behaviors, the media and advertising have the potential to contribute to the creation of an environment that is supportive. Media activities that are responsible have the potential to combat negative cultural norms and contribute to the development of a culture that places a high priority on overall well-being.

To summarize, the process of constructing communities that are supportive requires the active participation of individuals such as family members, friends, healthcare professionals, workplaces, educational institutions, and mainstream media. By contributing to an environment in which individuals feel encouraged, inspired, and empowered to make and maintain positive choices for their weight management and overall well-being, these entities contribute to the creation of favorable conditions.

CHAPTER 12

A FUTURE OF HOPE AND INNOVATION

An exciting and innovative future is emerging in the field of obesity prevention and treatment, which is being driven by cutting-edge research and technological developments. This future is filled with optimism and innovation.

A deep dive into the complexities of genomics is being undertaken by researchers in order to identify the genetic markers that contribute to obesity. The results of this investigation set the groundwork for personalized medicine, which is a form of medical treatment in which actions can be precisely matched to the genetic profile of an individual. The ever-increasing comprehension of the influences of genetics holds the potential to bring forth treatments that are more efficient and specific.

The field of precision nutrition is gaining popularity as it makes use of insights into the specific dietary requirements, metabolic processes, and gut microbiota of an individual. In order to facilitate the development of personalized dietary advice, the relationship between diet and the microbiota in the gut is becoming increasingly transparent. In order to improve gut health and tackle the issue of obesity on a molecular level, this individualized nutritional approach is being used.

Personal health monitoring and management are undergoing a transformation as a result of the proliferation of wearable technologies, such as fitness trackers and smartwatches. Providing users with real-time data on their food habits, patterns of physical activity, and sleep patterns enables them to make more educated decisions. Through the use of digital health platforms, engagement is increased, and chances for continual support and feedback are made available.

Telemedicine is bringing about a revolution in the delivery of healthcare, particularly in the context of the management of obesity. The use of remote monitoring and virtual consultations makes it possible for healthcare providers to provide patients with continuing assistance and to help them through the process of managing their weight more effectively. This strategy improves accessibility and overcomes potential obstacles that may prevent patients from receiving care in person.

Bariatric surgery, which is an essential component in the treatment of severe obesity, is continuously undergoing development with the introduction of new methods and technology. Surgical interventions are becoming more effective and safer as a result of the development of novel technologies, robotic-assisted surgery, and minimally invasive treatments. These advancements can open up new opportunities for individuals who could potentially benefit from these procedures.

Recent developments in the field of neuroscience are improving our understanding of the intricate brain networks that control behavior and appetite. Brain stimulation techniques, such as deep brain stimulation and transcranial magnetic stimulation, are currently being investigated as potential tools for modulating these circuits. This presents a novel opportunity for the intervention of obesity.

The landscape of pharmacotherapy is evolving, and researchers are creating drugs that target specific pathways related to the regulation of hunger and the metabolism of energy. These drugs, when paired with treatments that focus on lifestyle, present a multidimensional approach to the management and loss of weight.

The fields of artificial intelligence and machine learning are making important contributions by analyzing enormous datasets in order to recognize trends and improve predictive models. The application of these technologies has the potential to improve our understanding of the factors that contribute to obesity, the responses to therapy, and the outcomes, which will ultimately result in interventions that are more accurate and successful.

The convergence of research and technology offers a future in which obesity prevention and treatment will become increasingly personalized, comprehensive, and impactful. This is a landscape that is filled with hope and creativity. Individuals who are attempting to navigate the complexity of obesity and are working towards healthier lives have a better chance of success if they continue to pursue education and incorporate technological tools into their lives.

CHAPTER 13

MOVING FORWARD

Together, let us embrace a message of optimism and empowerment as we go forward on the path of solving the issue of obesity. Every single person holds the ability to bring about positive change and the power to steer their own health and well-being in the right direction.

It is not about reaching perfection but rather making progress on the route to healthier living. Small, long-term adjustments to one's nutrition, level of physical activity, and mental attitude can have a significant impact over the course of time. It is a voyage of self-discovery, of understanding what works specifically for each individual, and of discovering joy in the process throughout the journey.

It is important to keep in mind that failures are an inevitable component of any transforming journey. The most important thing is to have the ability to recover quickly from setbacks, gain wisdom from experiences, and continue going forward. A mindset of self-compassion should be cultivated, and every accomplishment, no matter how insignificant it may seem, should be celebrated, because they all add to the bigger tapestry of positive transformation.

You should surround yourself with a community that is supportive, whether it be friends, family, or experts in the healthcare field. Encouragement should be sought out, goals should be shared, and strength should be drawn from individuals who inspire and motivate you. We have the ability to work together to create surroundings that encourage healthy choices and overall well-being.

The power of individual agency in making choices based on information should be acknowledged. As a result of gaining an awareness of one's own preferences, establishing goals that are attainable, and incorporating activities that provide pleasure into one's daily routine, good change becomes not only attainable but also sustainable. One has the potential to make an investment in their own health and future well-being with every decision one makes.

The idea of holistic health should be embraced, and it should be acknowledged that well-being involves not only the physical but also the mental and emotional elements. Make self-care a top priority, cultivate positivity in your relationships, and engage in mindfulness practices. It is possible to live a life that is both healthier and more fulfilling by adopting a balanced approach that places priority on total wellness.

With regard to this voyage, there is no answer that is universally applicable. At the same time that every person is one of a kind, the pursuit of health is an endeavor that is intensely personal. By arming yourself with knowledge, seeking help when it is required, and having faith in your ability to make decisions that are in line with your well-being, you can empower yourself.

The foreseeable future is replete with possibilities for effecting constructive change. Let us embark on this road with the notion that each step forward is a step towards a life that is healthier and more vibrant. With hope serving as our compass and empowerment serving as our guide, let us do so with determination, resilience, and the conviction that each stride forward is a step towards a life that is more flourishing.

SELF REFLECTION QUESTIONS

1 What changes have occurred in my comprehension of obesity as a result of my exposure to the several definitions and classifications of the condition?

2 What can I learn about the magnitude of this problem and the sense of urgency it carries from the worldwide burden of obesity?

3 Have I discovered any personal risk factors for obesity in my own life, based on my food, my level of physical activity, or any other aspects?

4 What are my thoughts on the impact that social and environmental factors have on the level of weight management that an individual achieves?

5 To what extent do I believe that genetic predisposition plays a part in obesity, and how does this influence my perspective on the responsibility that I have for my own actions?

6. Have I given any thought to the potential negative effects that obesity could have on my own physical and mental health as well as the health of others around me?

7. What are my thoughts on the role that prejudice and stigma play in people's perceptions of obesity in society? When I first learned about the relationship between obesity and other health problems, what was the most surprising thing to me?

8. Which of my own ideas about healthy eating is most important to me, and how can I incorporate those beliefs into my own dietary decisions?

9. What are some of the practical ways that I might overcome obstacles to engaging in regular physical activity, and what are some of the things that encourage me to go?

10. To what extent am I willing to investigate various approaches to weight management, including behavioral and psychological methods?

11. Which public health and policy initiatives do I believe have the potential to be the most effective in combating the epidemic of obesity?

12. What are some ways that I can help develop communities that are supportive, encourage healthy behaviors, and fight against the stigma associated with weight?

To what extent do I agree or disagree with the ethical considerations that are associated with obesity research and treatment?

13. What adjustments am I prepared to undertake in my own life in order to encourage better behaviors and contribute to a solution?

14. What strategies can I use to successfully advocate for improved policies and resources to combat obesity on a societal and neighborhood level?

15. What message of optimism and resiliency do I want to convey to others as we continue our fight against obesity?

The questions presented here are merely a starting point; you are free to modify or build upon them in accordance with your particular experiences and areas of interest. It is important to keep in mind that self-reflection is an ongoing process and that returning to these questions throughout the course of your reading can offer you significant insights and give you the ability to take action.

www.ingramcontent.com/pod-product-compliance
Lightning Source LLC
Chambersburg PA
CBHW070731260726
48660CB00007B/2788